Boys and Girls

Brushing Your Teeth Is Fun

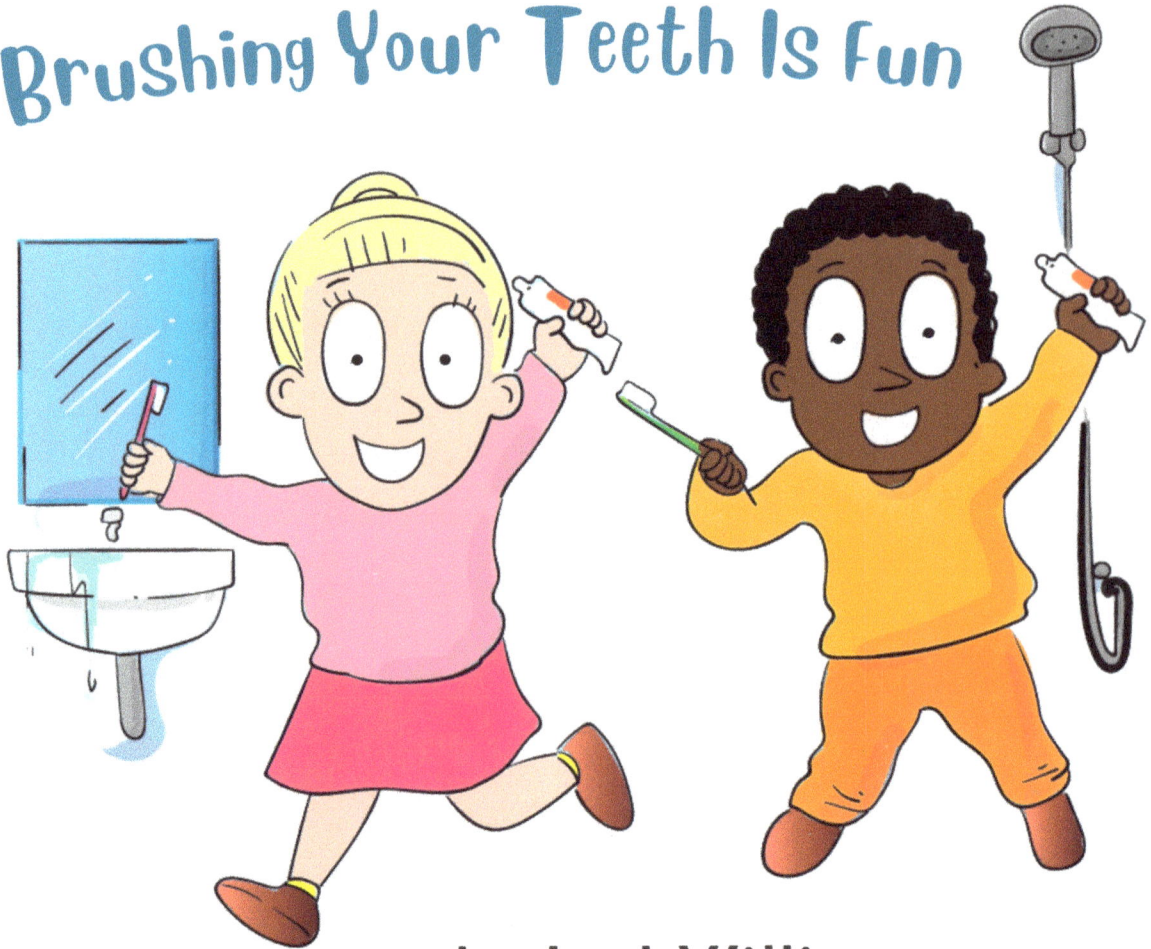

by Inel Williams

Boys and girls,
brushing your teeth is fun!
But how do we get it done?

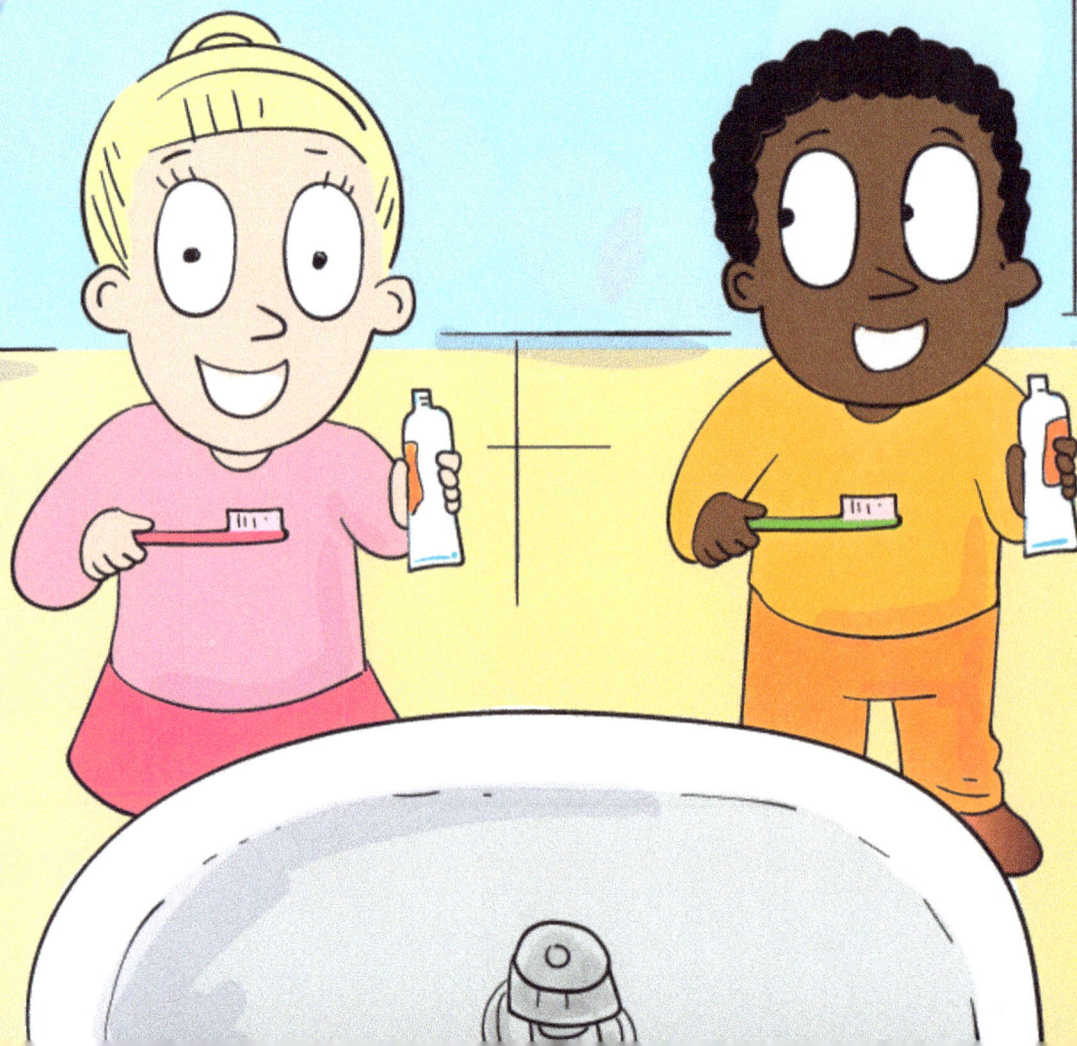

Here are 5 rules for you to follow:

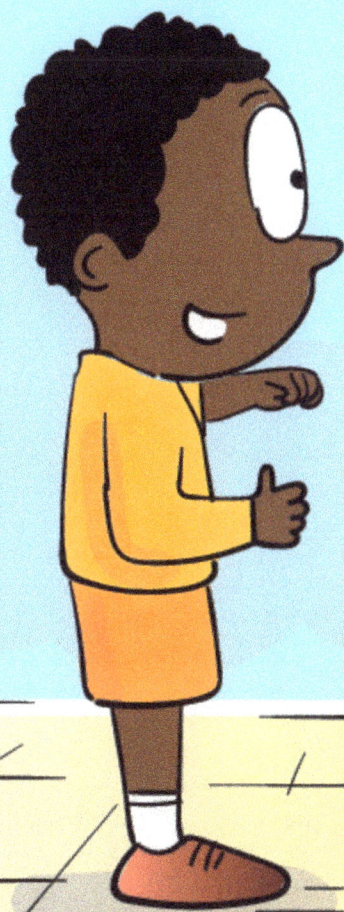

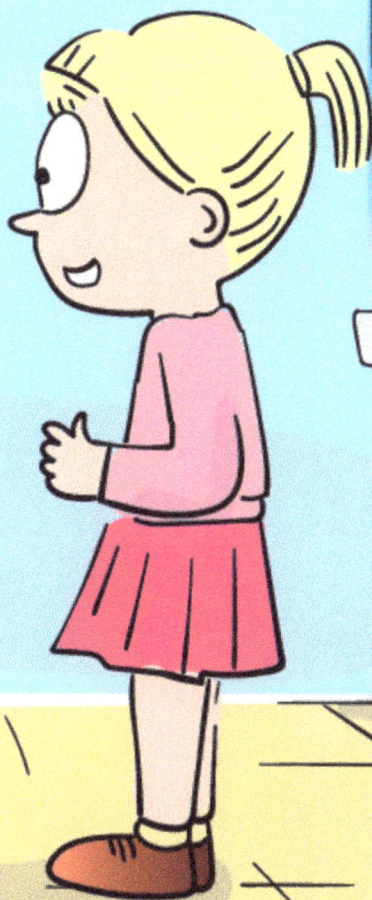

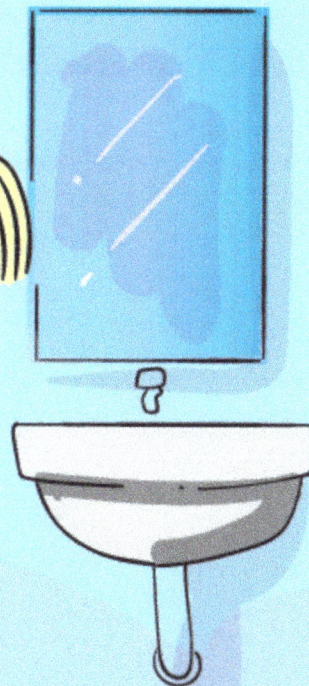

When it comes to toothpaste,
rule number 1: don't swallow!

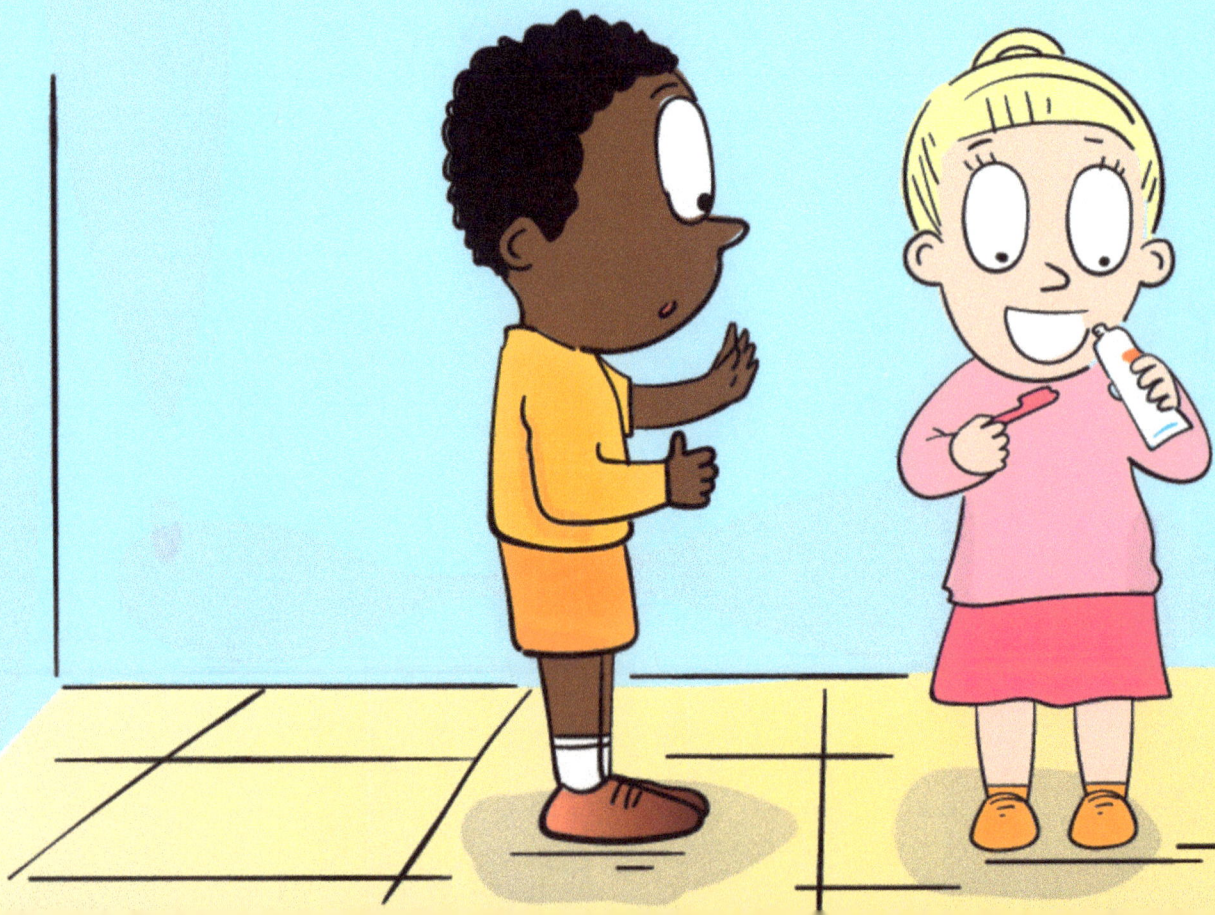

Rule number 2: don't use too much,

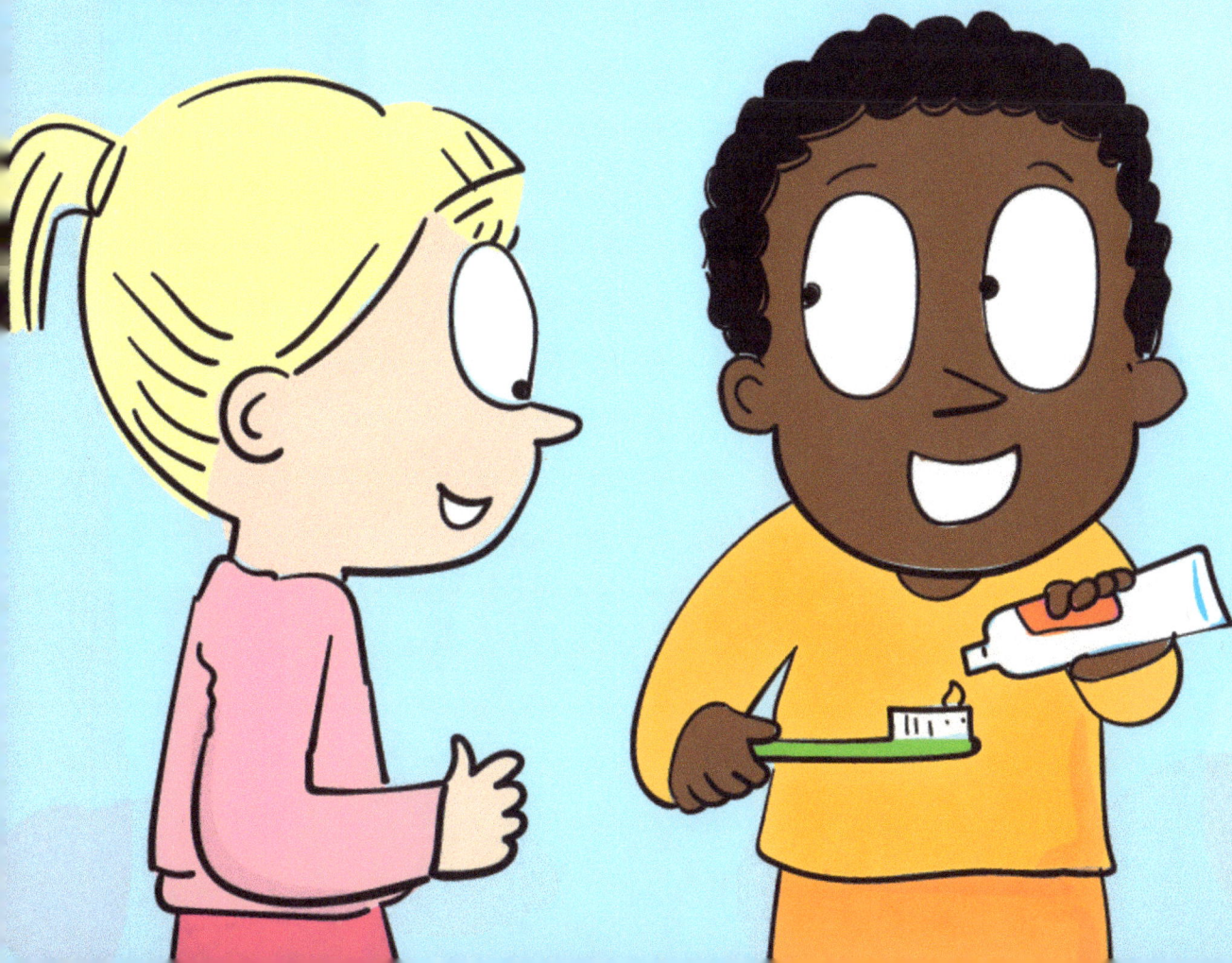

you don't need a lot on your brush.

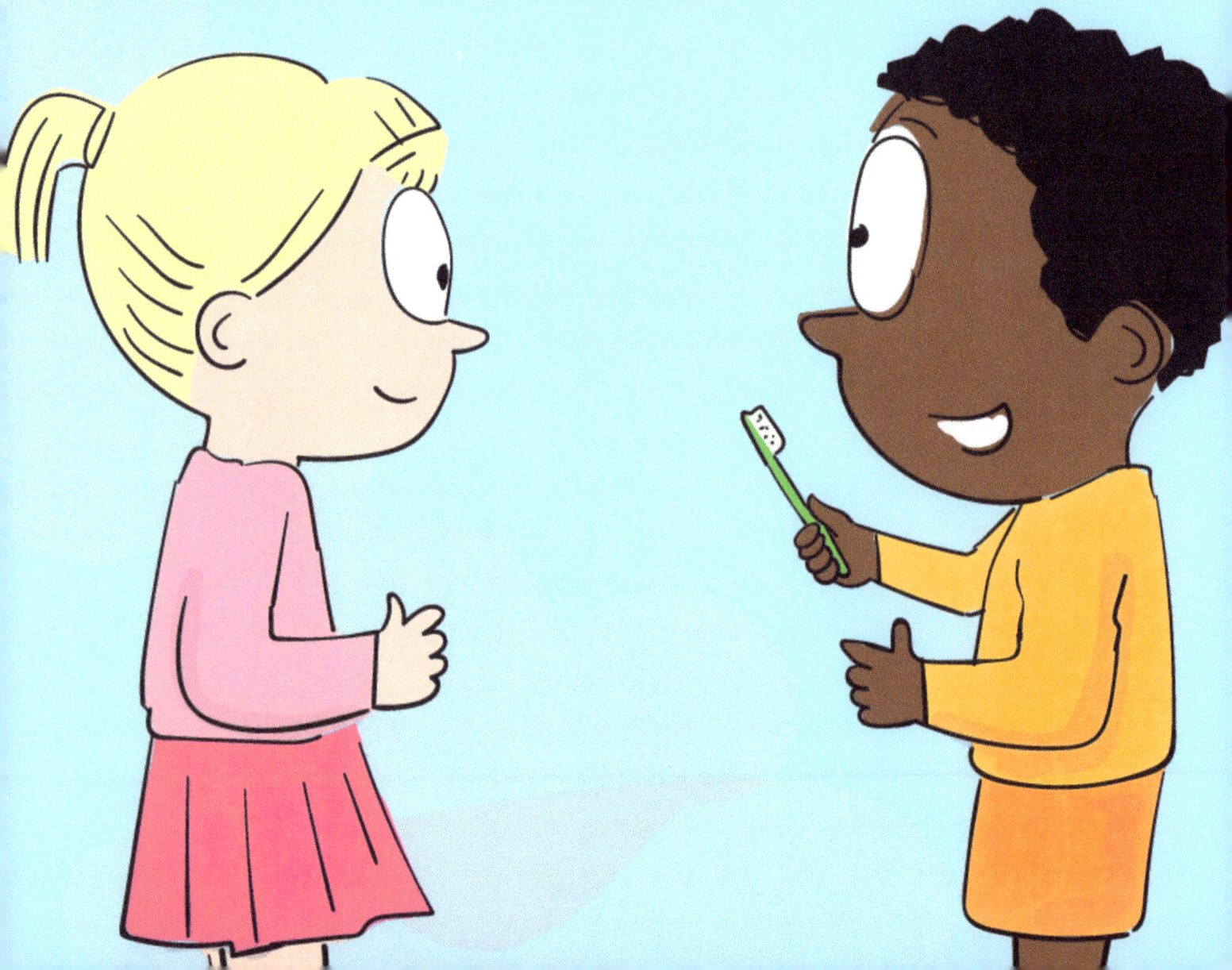

Use an amount the size of 1 pea,

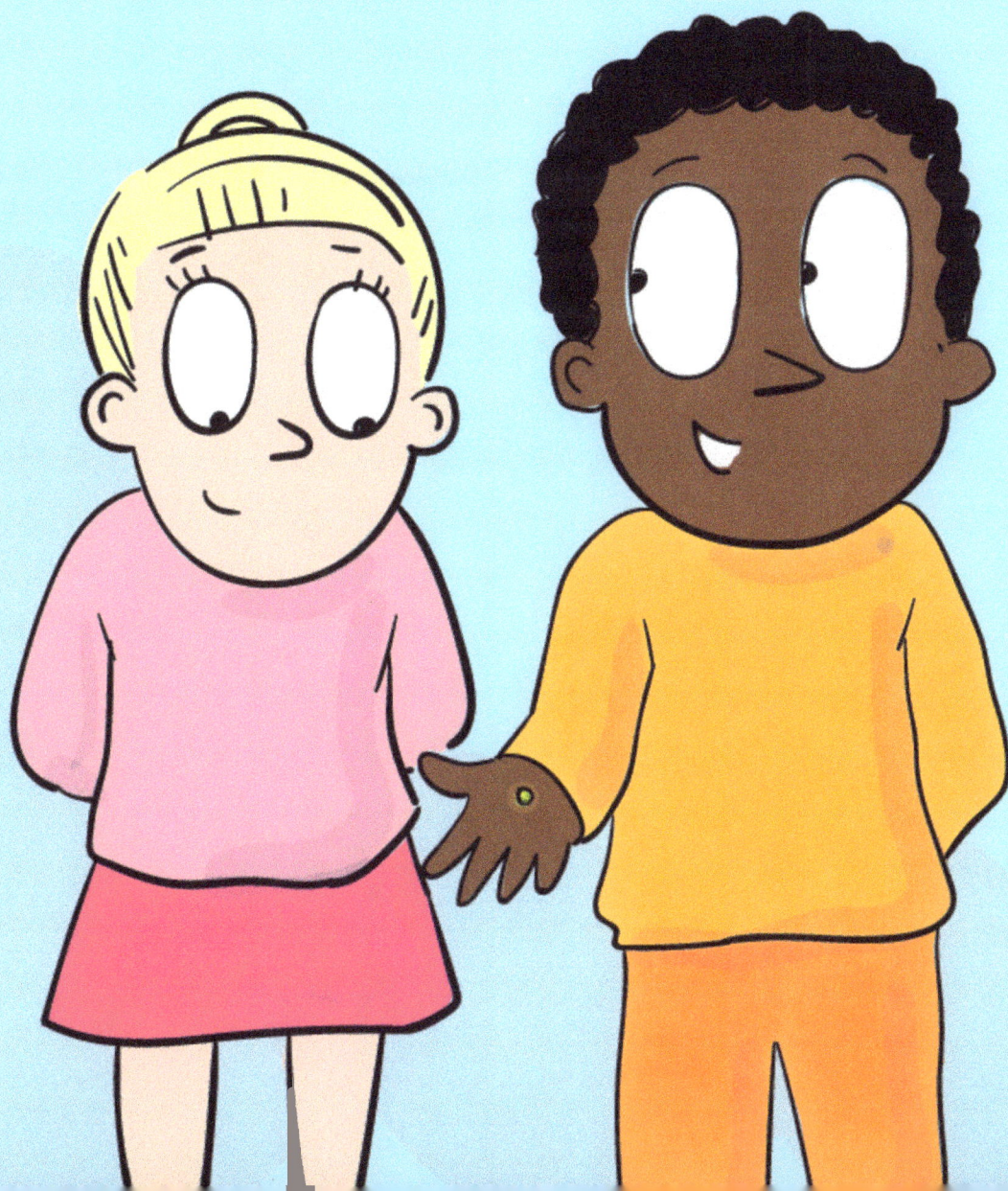

it's better than too much,
don't you agree?

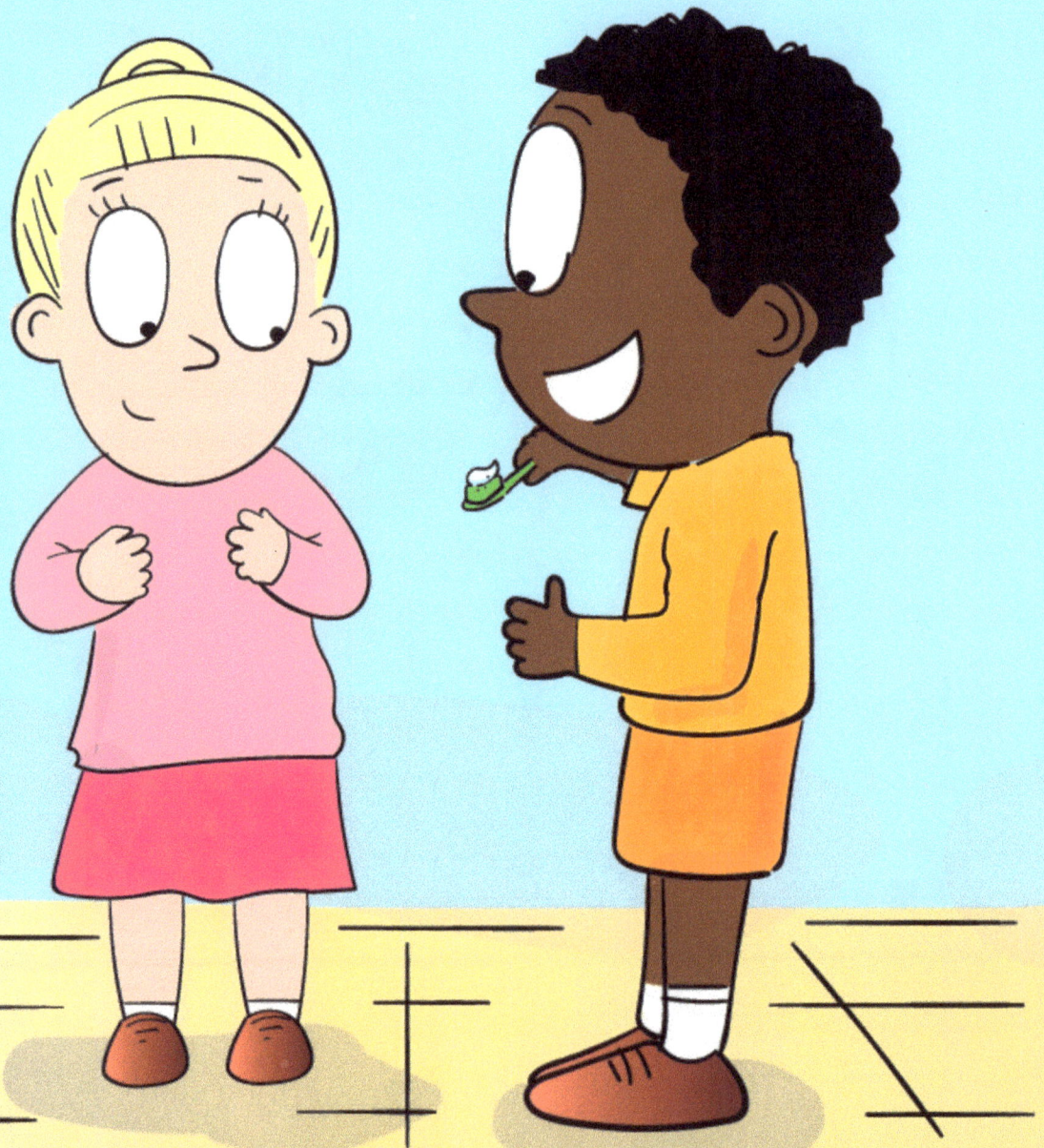

Take your brush with toothpaste
and then put it in place

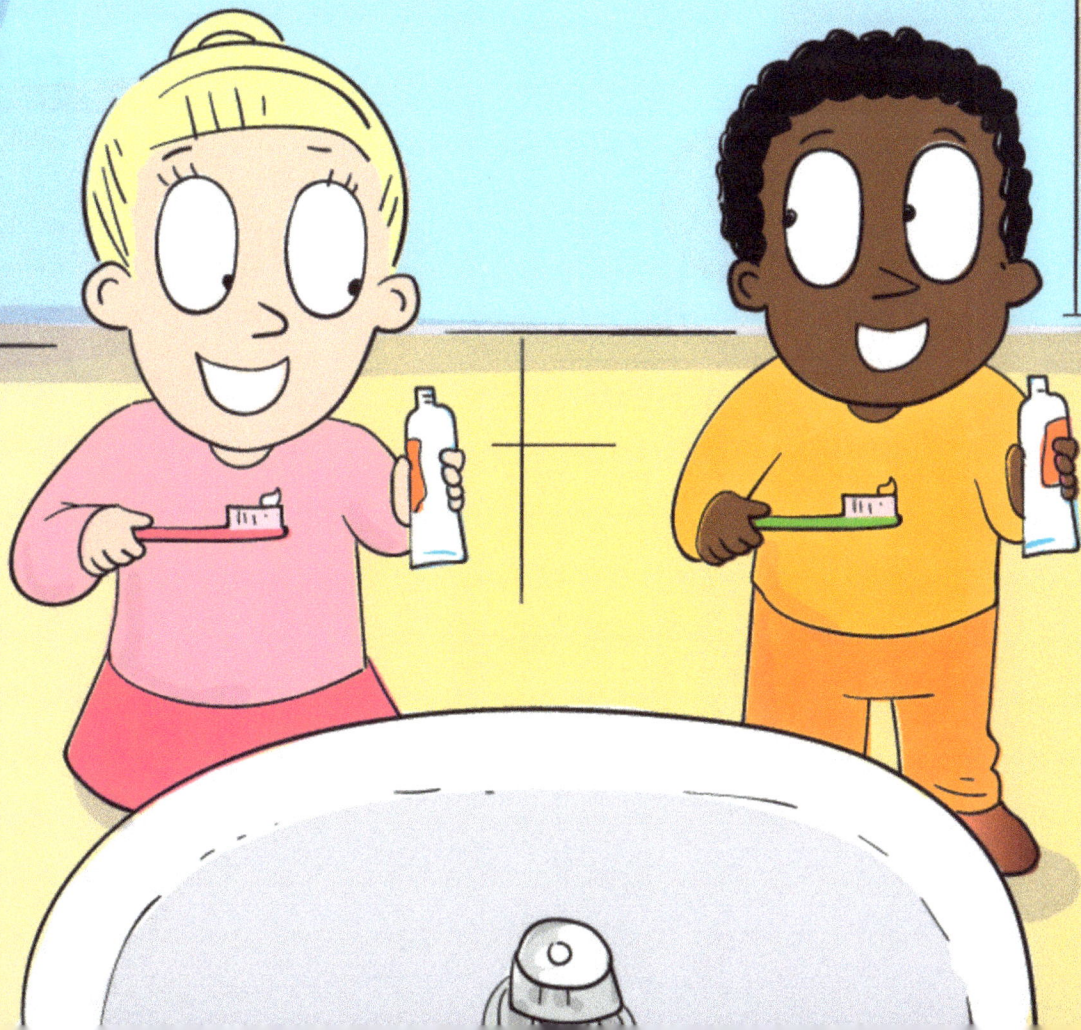

in your mouth, on your teeth,
to clean up all the food you eat.

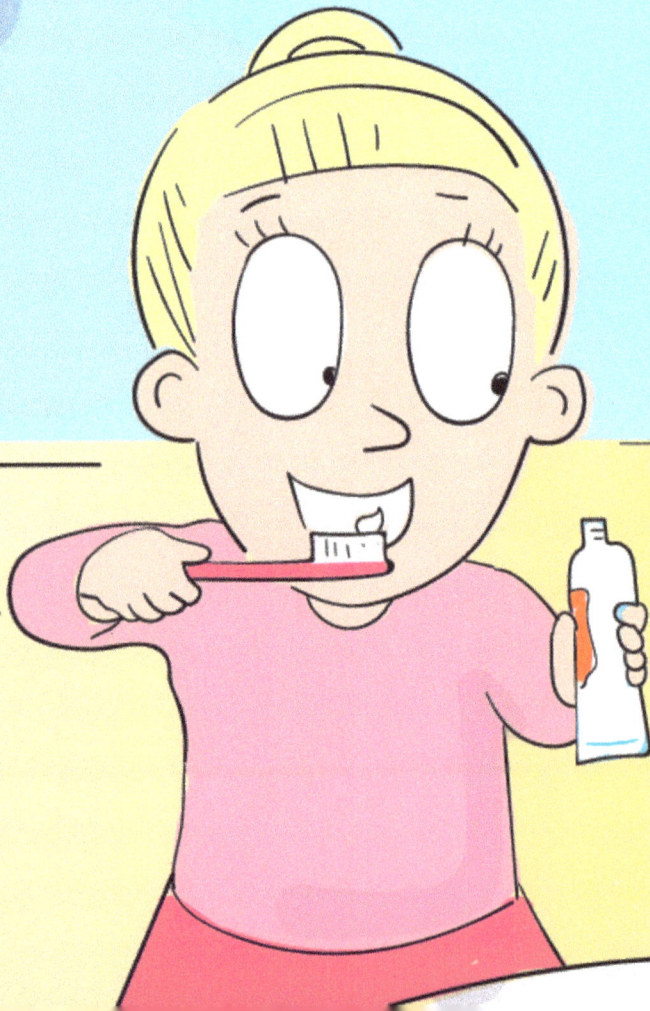

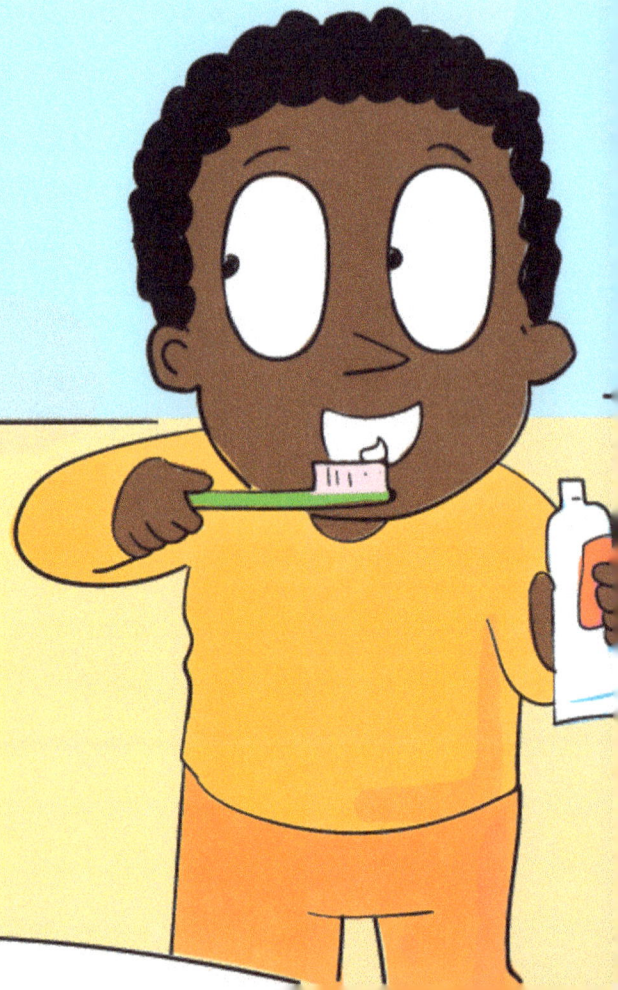

On your front teeth you start
moving your brush around...

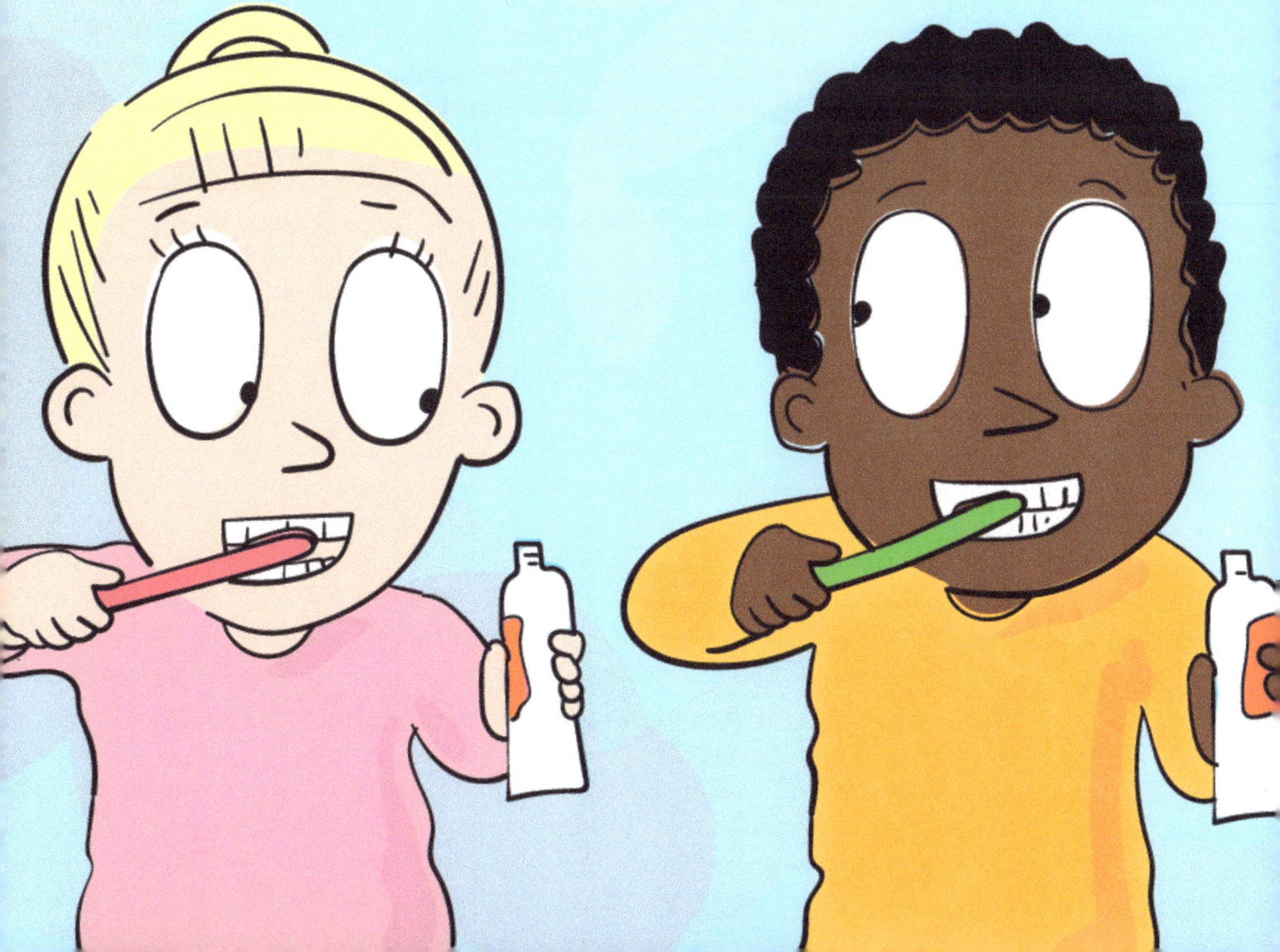

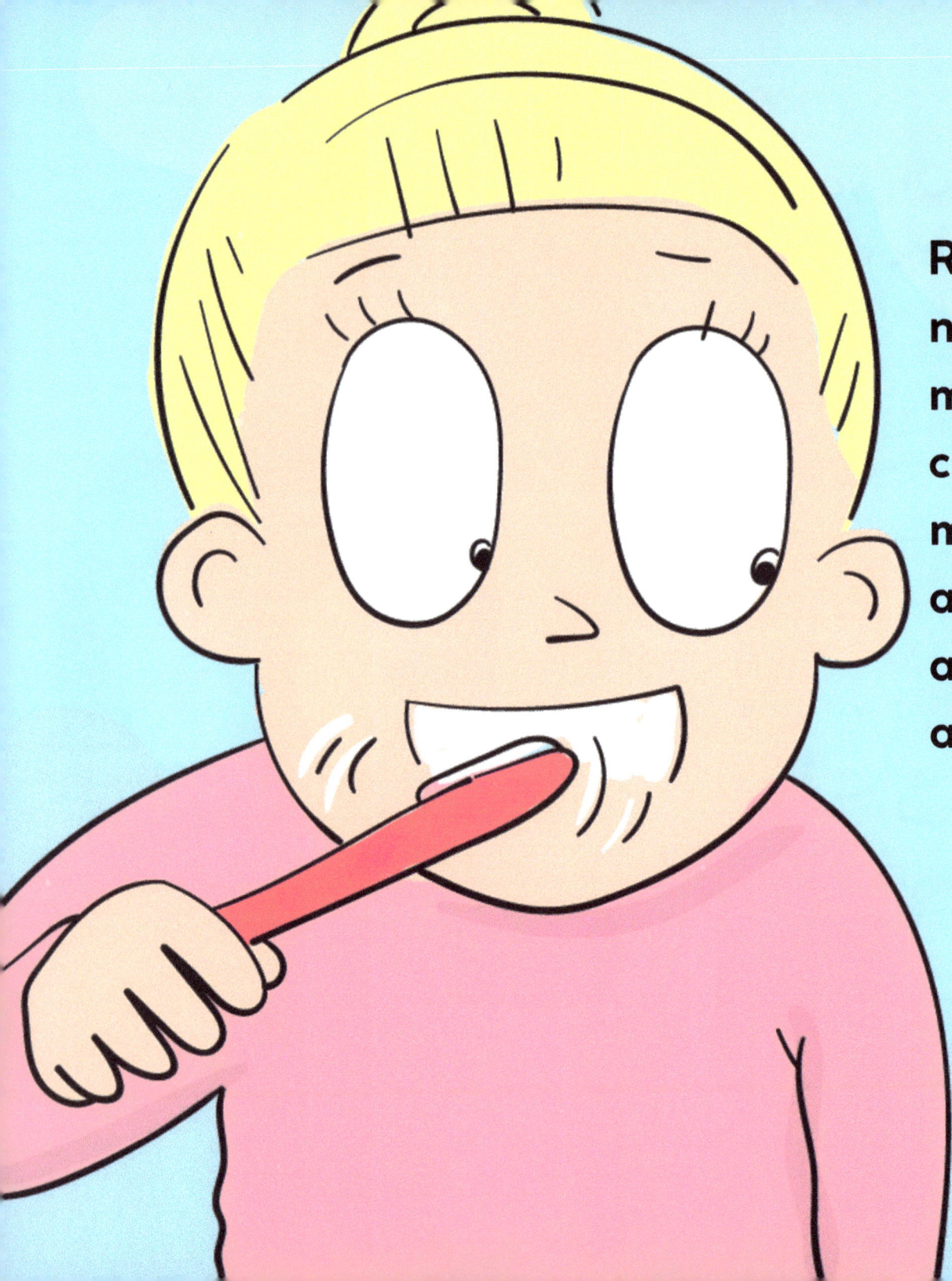

Rule number 3: move it in circles, then move back and forth, and up and down.

And then
you brush
your teeth
in the back.

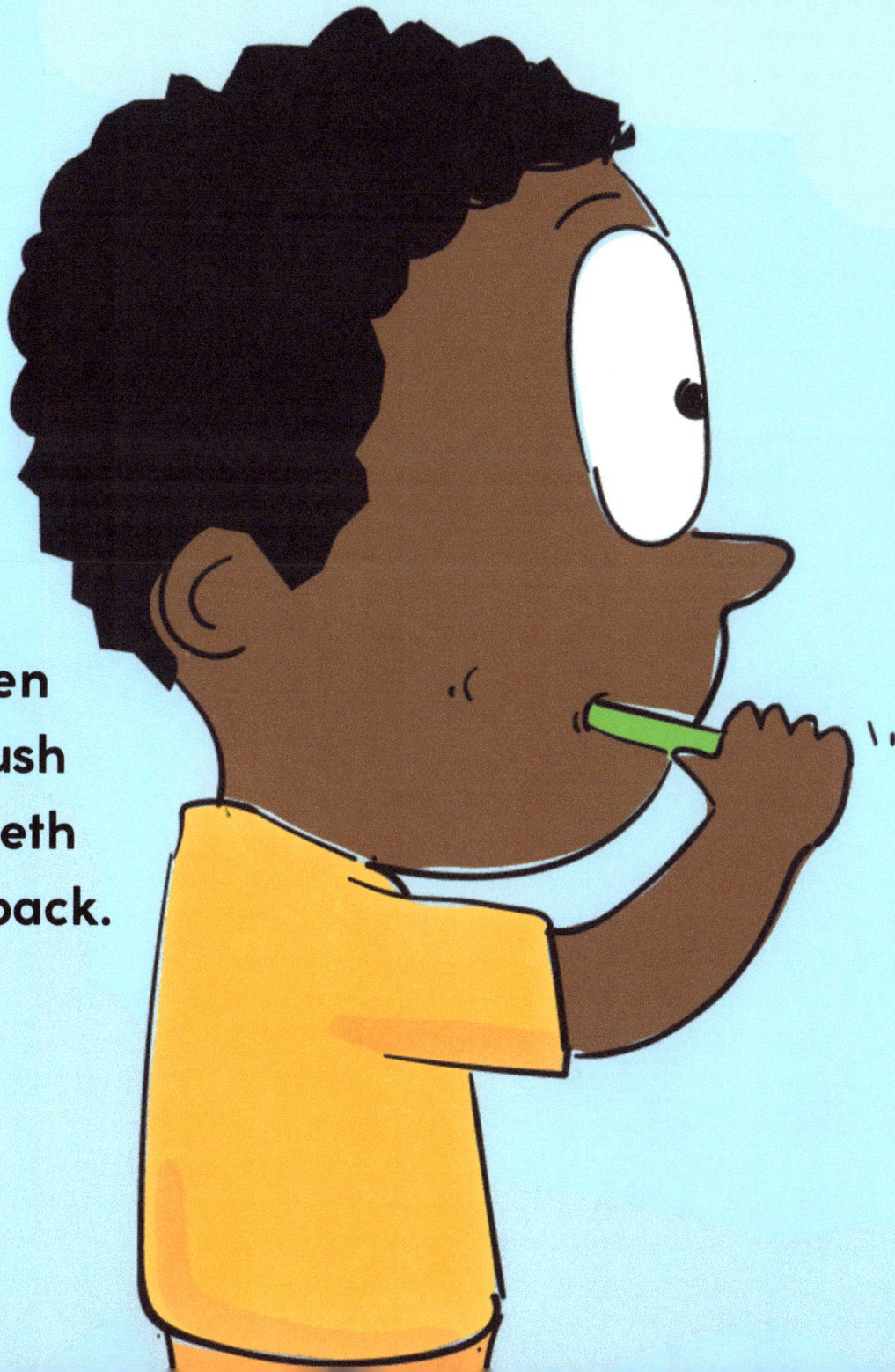

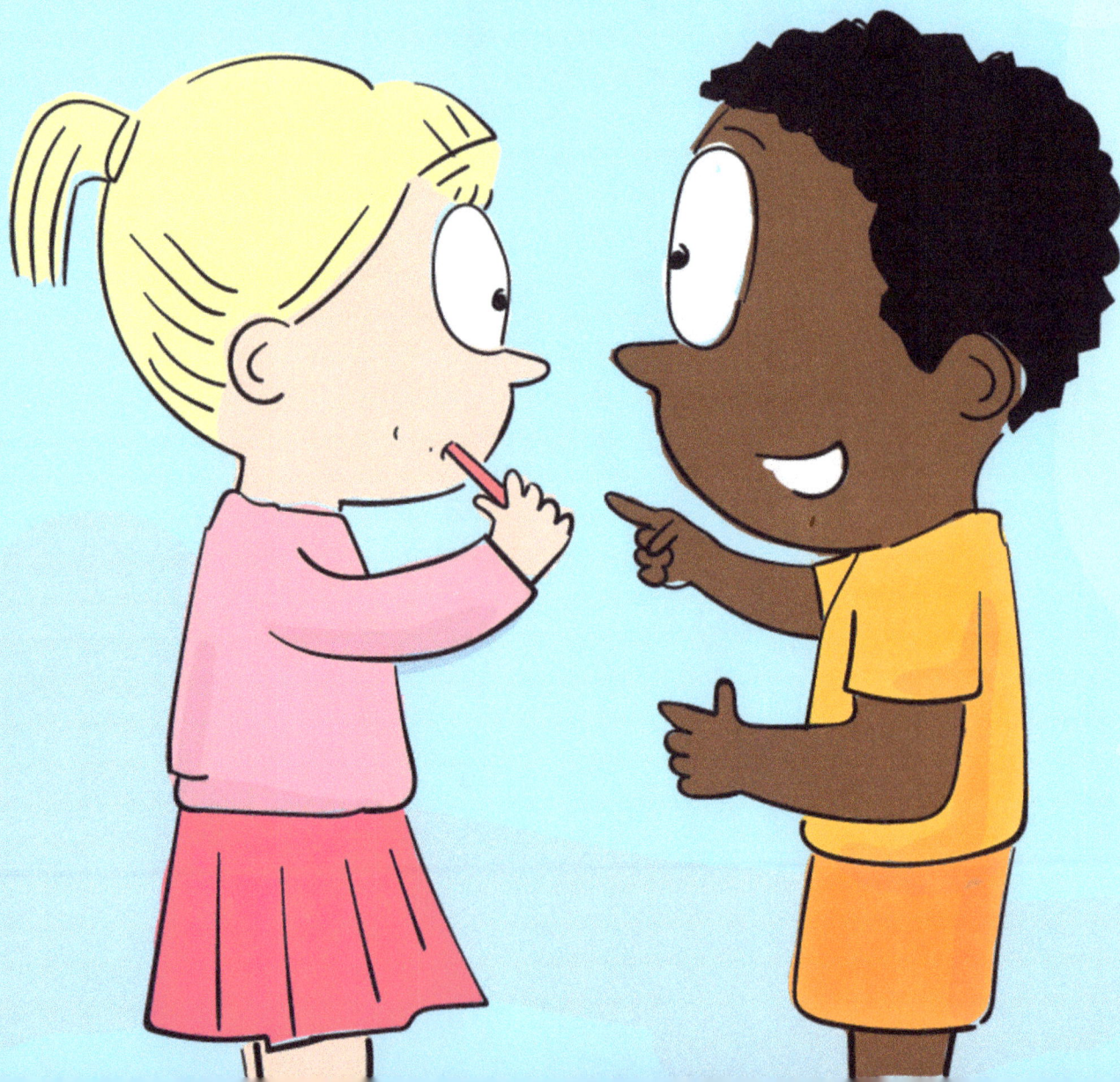

If you don't, you might get plaque!

And if you don't want your breath to smell

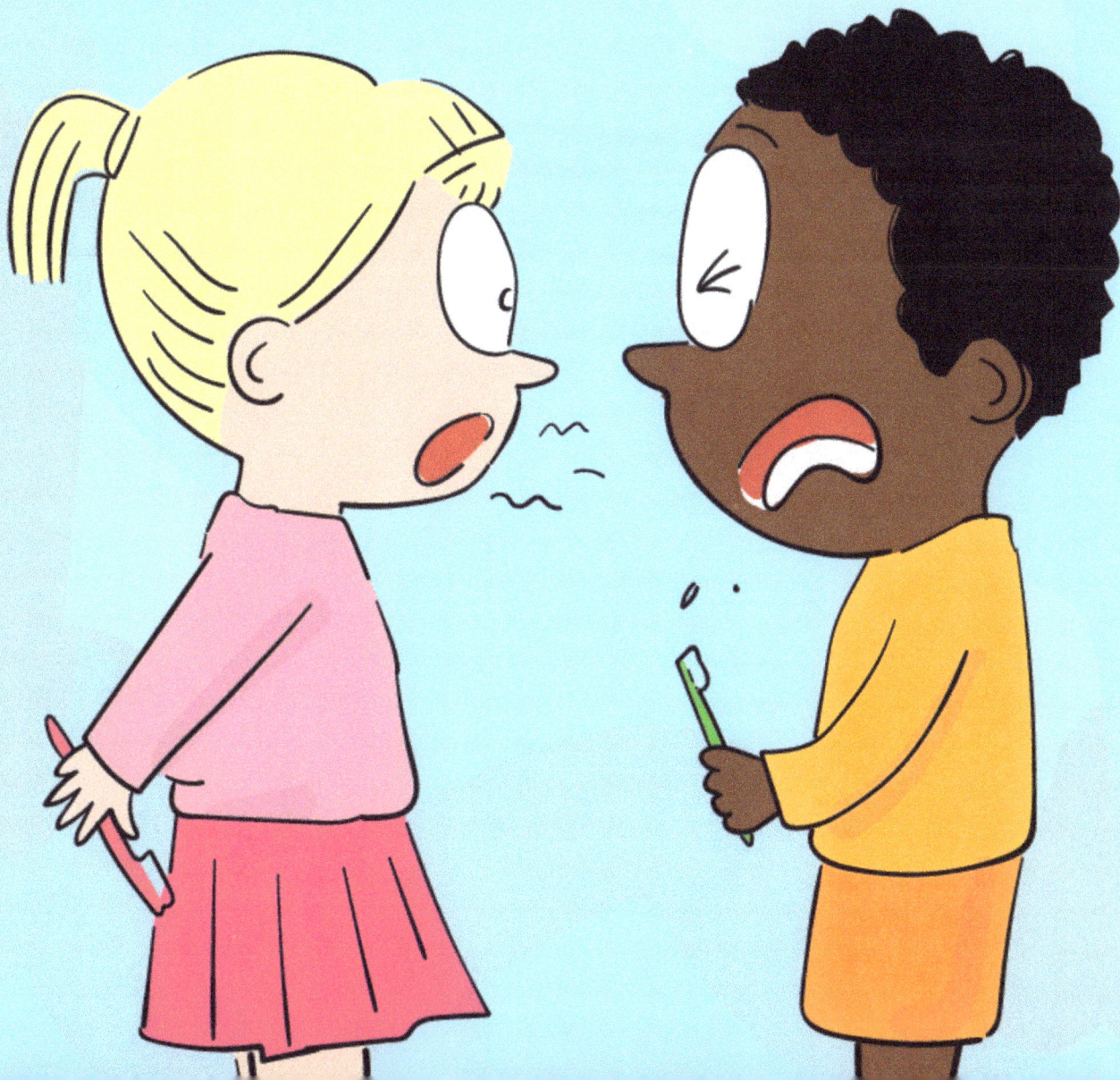

don't forget your tongue!
Try to brush it well.

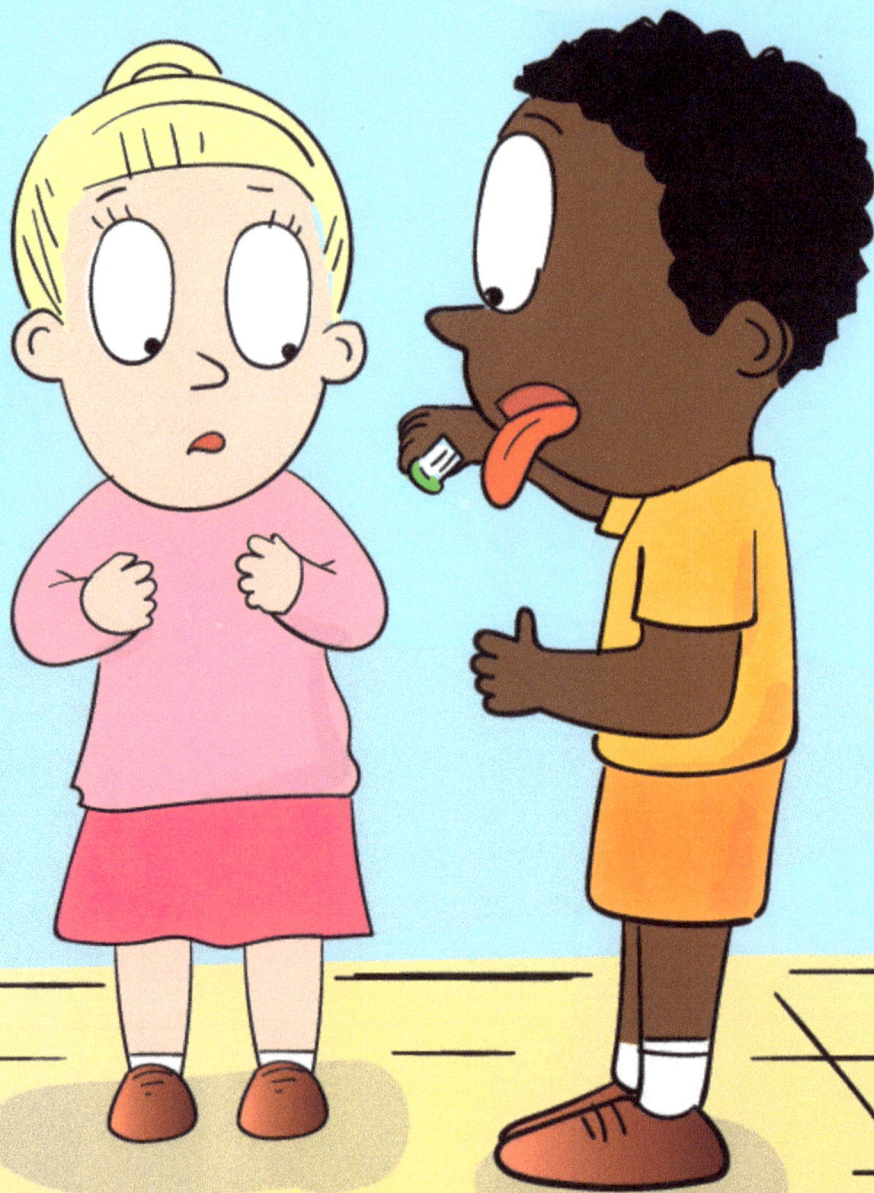

Brush your tongue back and forth,
and brush it up and down,

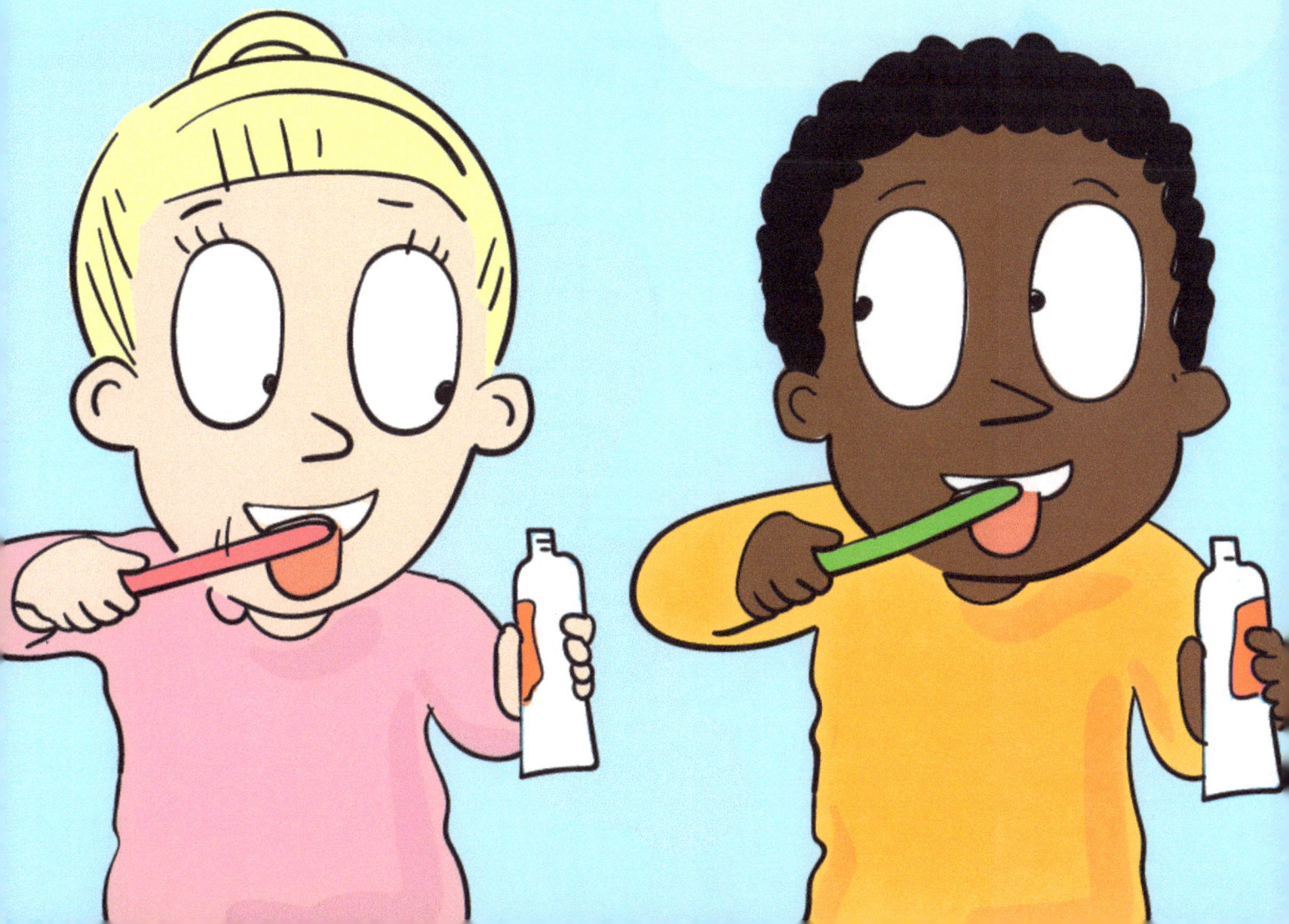

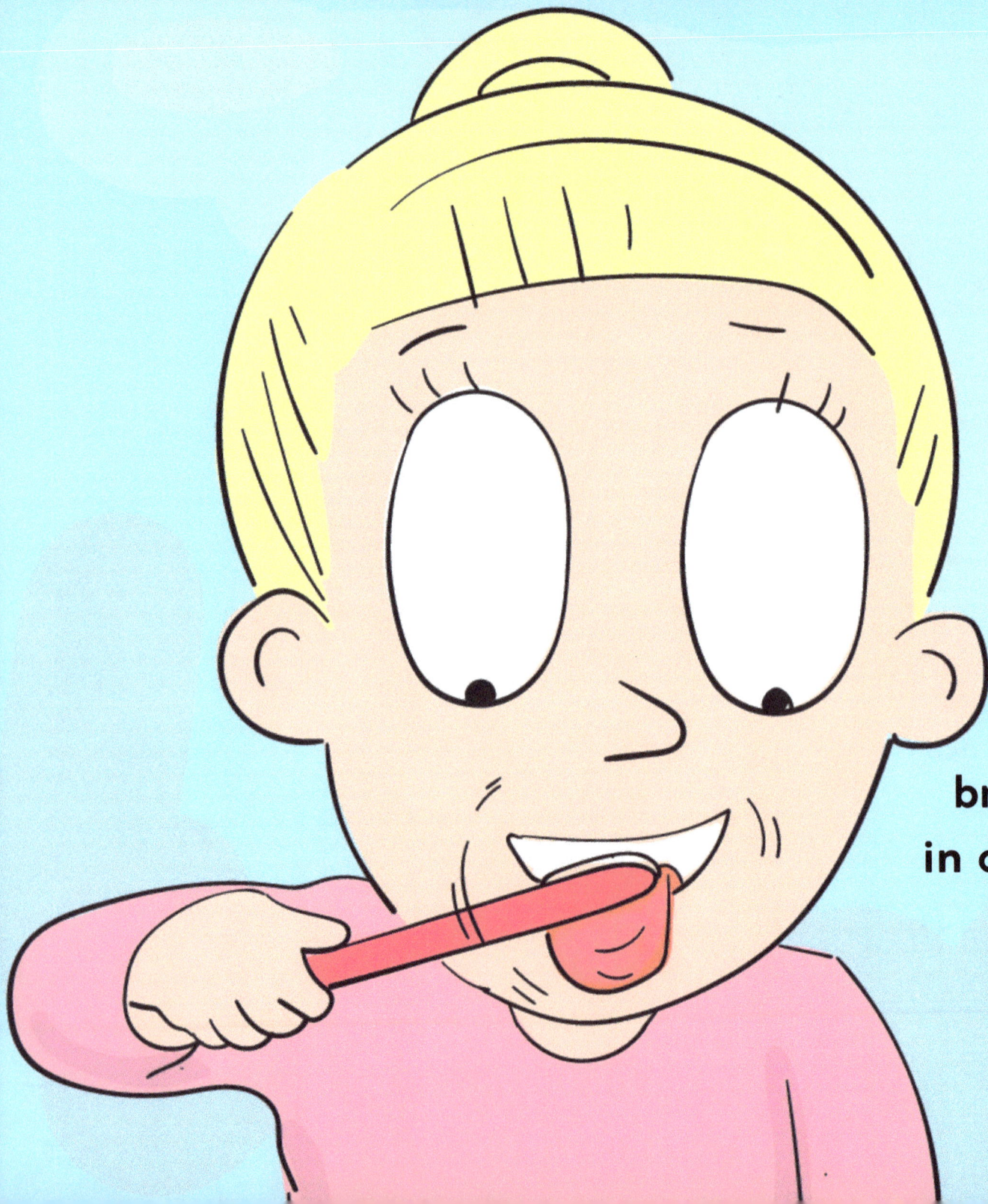

and
brush it
in circles
going
round
and
round.

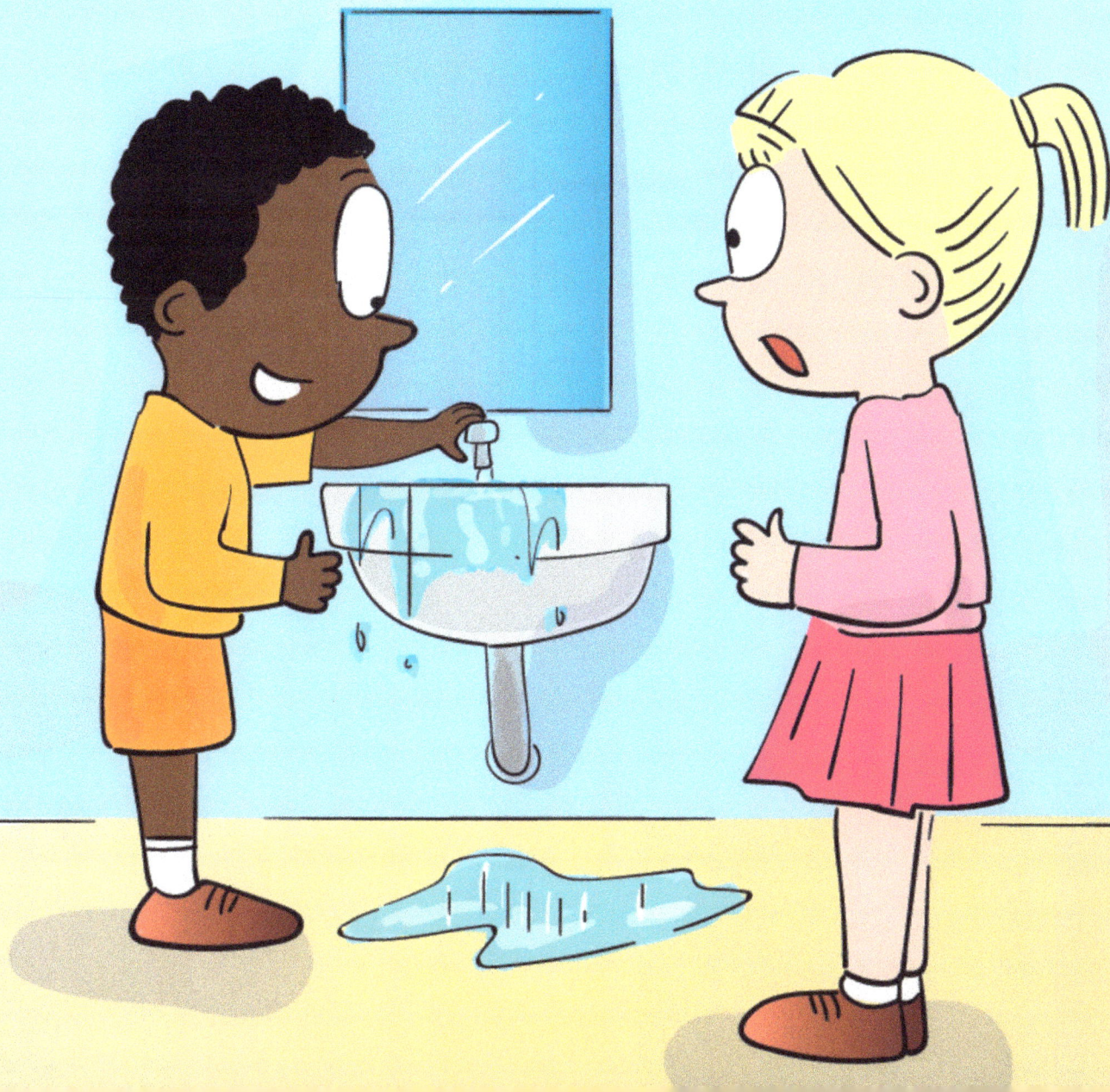
Rule number 4:
while you brush, don't run the water.

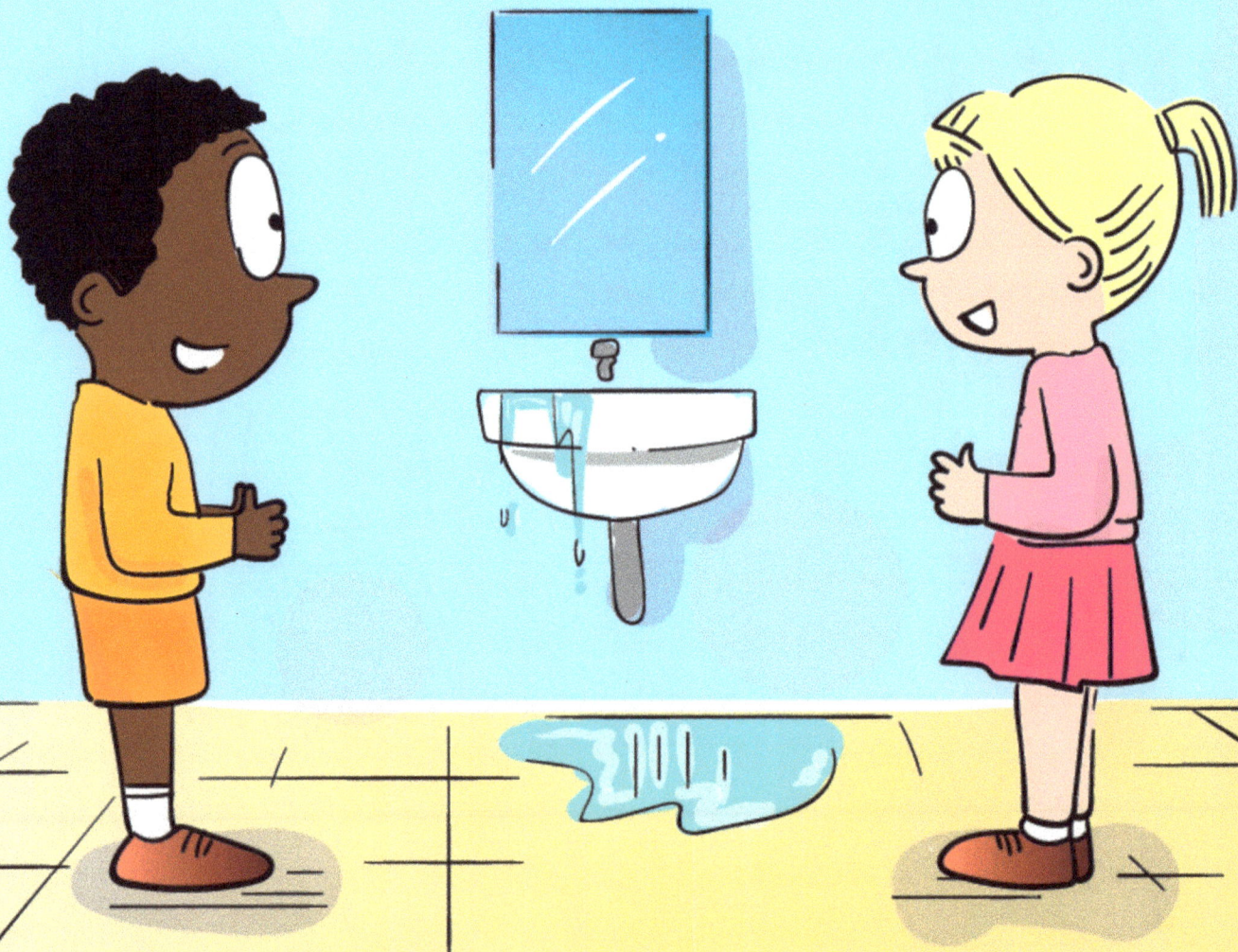

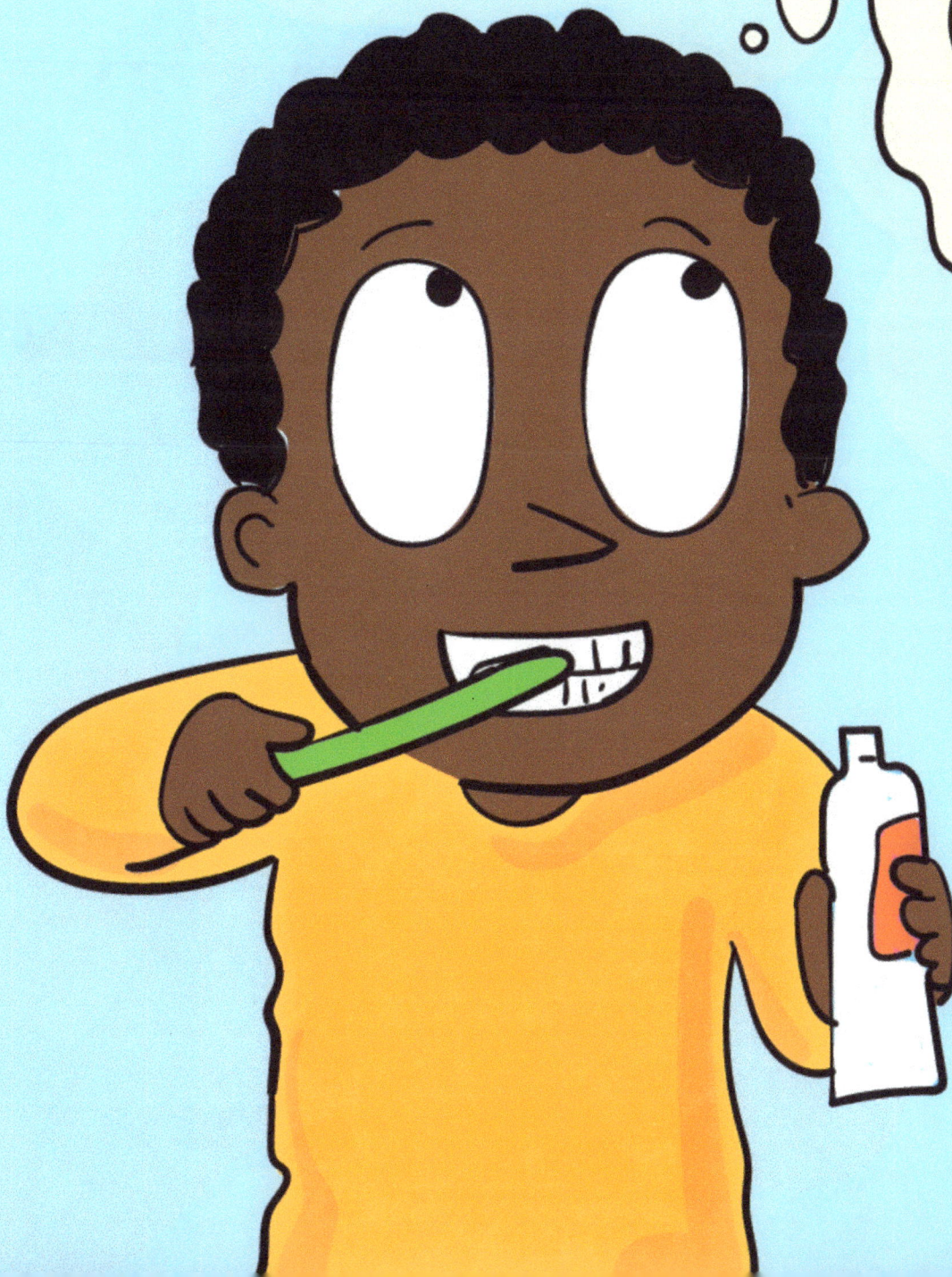

Also, while you have the chance...

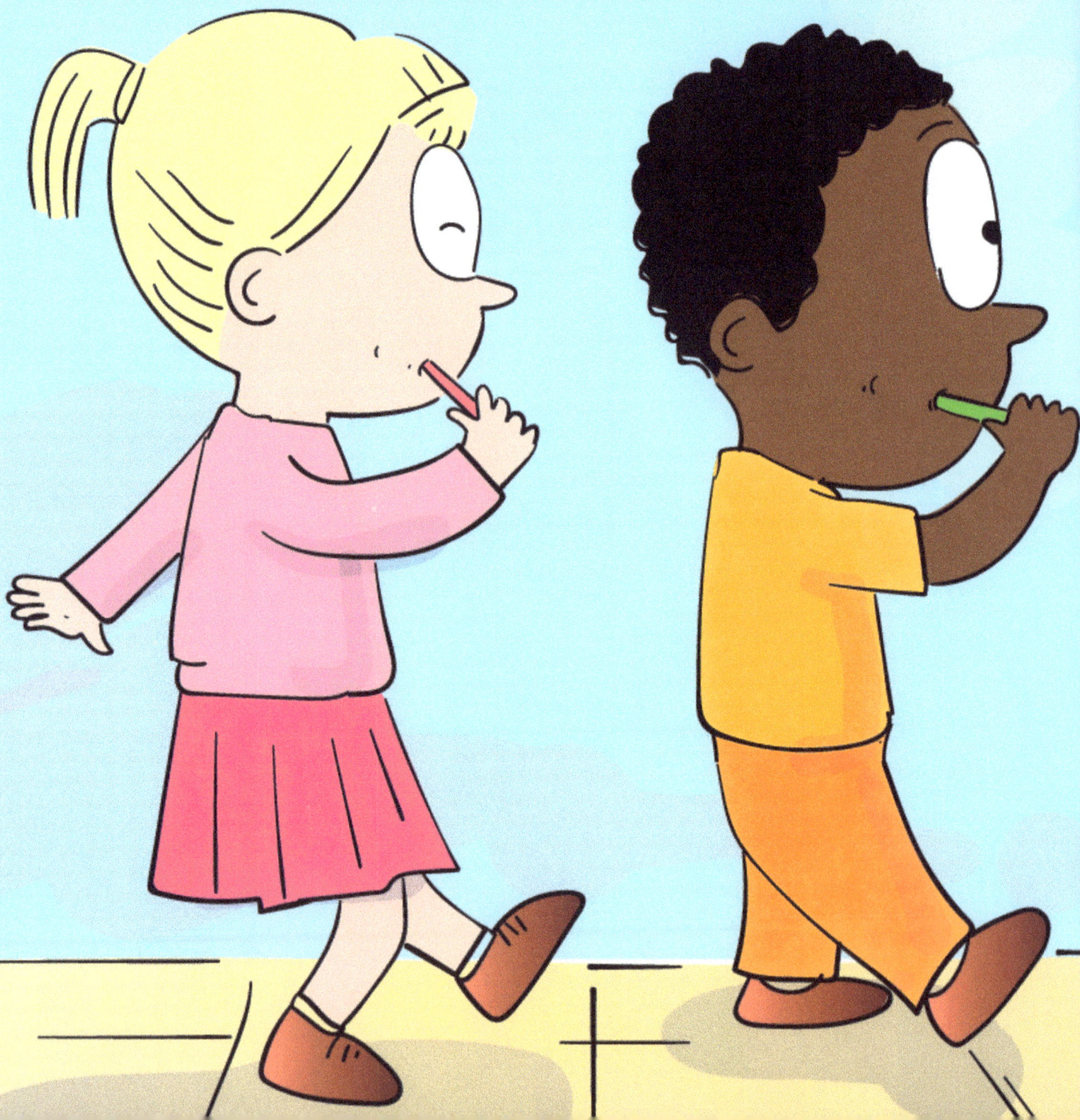

...as you brush your teeth, do a dance!

Rule number 5: don't forget hun
to wash your toothbrush
when you're done.

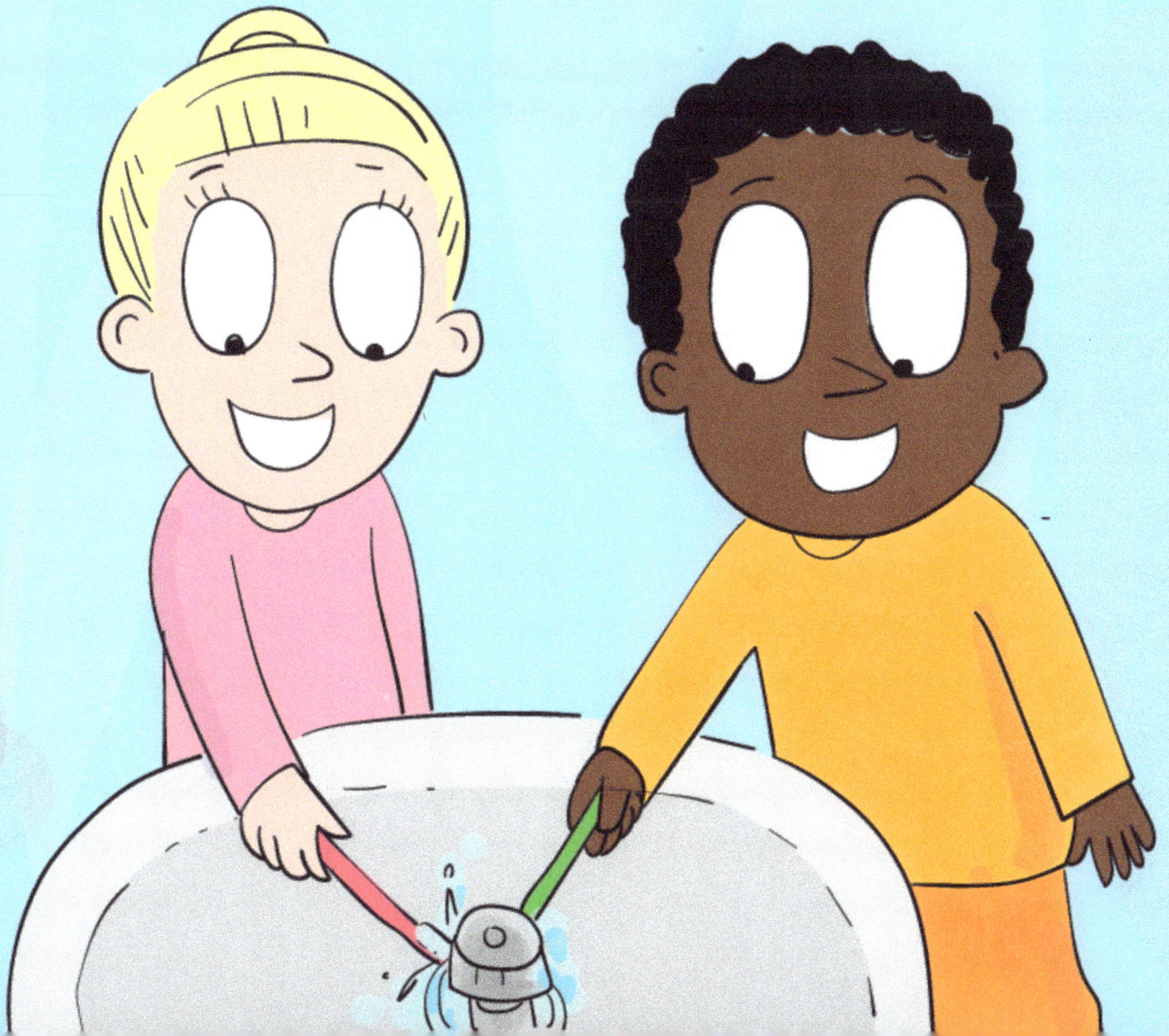

Now that all that fun is complete,
you now know how
to brush your teeth!

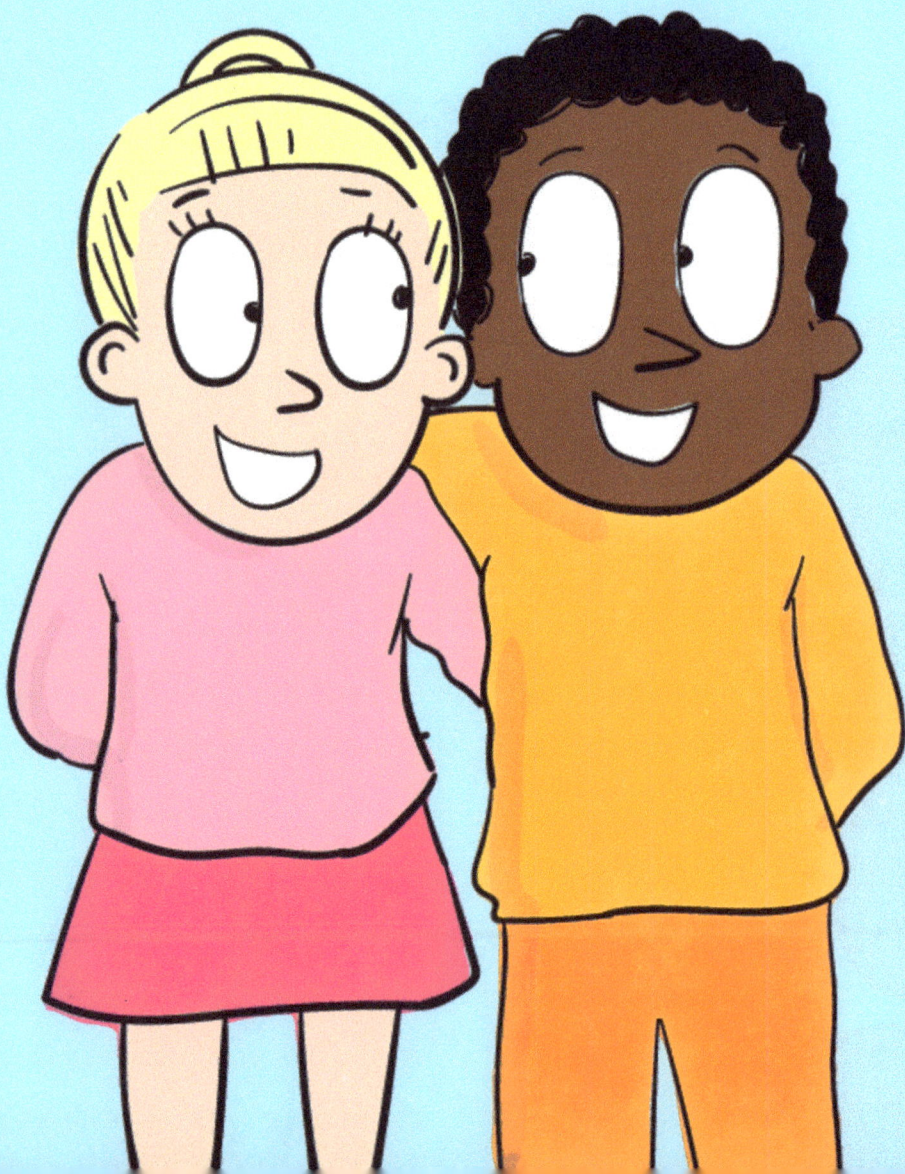

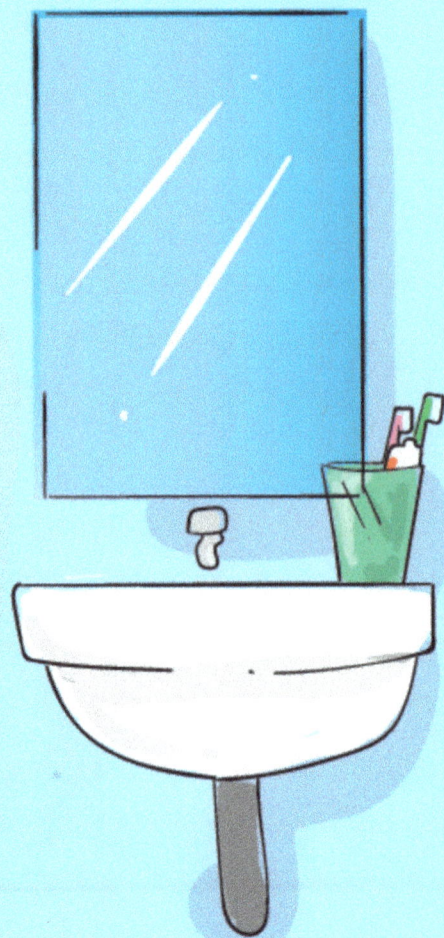

www.ingramcontent.com/pod-product-compliance
Lightning Source LLC
Chambersburg PA
CBHW041600260326
41914CB00011B/1327